Relapse Prevention
in Schizophrenia
and Other Psychoses

A treatment
workbook for the

Relapse Prevention in Schizophrenia and Other Psychoses

A treatment manual and
workbook for therapist and client

Dr John Sorensen

UNIVERSITY OF
HERTFORDSHIRE PRESS

First published in Great Britain in 2006 by
University of Hertfordshire Press
Learning and Information Services
University of Hertfordshire
College Lane
Hatfield
Hertfordshire AL10 9AB

British Library Cataloguing in Publication Data
A catalogue record for this book is available from the British Library

ISBN 1-902806-60-3 paperback manual plus 5 workbooks
ISBN 1-902806-61-1 pack of 10 workbooks sold separately

Design by Geoff Green Book Design, Cambridge CB4 5RA
Cover design by John Robertshaw, Harpenden AL5 2JB
Printed in Great Britain by Stephen Austin & Sons Ltd, Hertford SG13 7LU

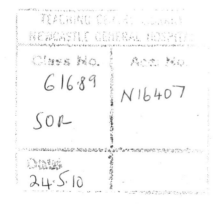

Imagination will beat its wings in vain
if we do not realise the necessity of
structural ascent. Build upwards
upon yesterday's experience.

*Ralph Maynard Smith (*The Ravine*)*

Contents

Acknowledgements

Special thanks go to the many clients who, over the years, have advised me on what has been helpful and less so in their treatment and interaction with services generally.

I would also like to thank Kathryn Smith without whose advice and editorial support the present manual would never have come about.

Dr John Sorensen
North Manchester General Hospital

Introduction

Since the publication of the original manual on *Relapse Prevention in Bipolar Disorder* (Sorensen, 2005) I have been approached by clients, parents, partners and clinicians working in the field, all asking me to adapt the original manual and treatment to psychosis in general and schizophrenia in particular. It appears that the format, style and simplicity of the manual have appealed to various interested groups and that the manual has been used in many ways since its recent publication. This interest, together with the positive feedback regarding the format and style of the intervention obtained from participants in the original research (Sorensen, Done and Rhodes, submitted), has caused me to agree to broaden the treatment's scope to encompass relapse prevention in psychosis generally.

The present treatment manual is the result of an extensive review of the relevant literature, conducted in order to adapt the bipolar manual to the needs of other client groups experiencing psychosis while retaining the characteristic style and 'flavour' of the original work. As such, the present manual has a different content, dealing with relapse prevention in schizophrenia and psychosis generally, but it has the style and format that some readers will recognise from the original bipolar manual which was so positively assessed by the participants who experienced it firsthand.

Psychosis and schizophrenia in particular can be, and frequently are, experienced as debilitating, recurring and severe mental illnesses, often occurring with serious secondary consequences such as suicidal behaviours, physical health problems, social disability and substance abuse (Blanchard, Brown, Horan and Sherwood, 2000; Hogarty and Flesher, 1999; Penn, Mueser, Spaulding, Hope and Reed, 1995; Rosenfarb, Nuechterlein, Goldstein and Subotnik, 2000; Tsuang, Wollson and Fleming, 1980; Wiersma, Nienhuis, Slooff and Giel, 1998). It is also clear that these problems are frequently confounded by impairments in occupational and social functioning more generally and that these impairments persist even between acute episodes of illness when symptom relief has been achieved for someone with relapsing or chronic schizophrenia or other psychosis (American Psychiatric Association, 1994; Johnstone, MacMillan, Frith, Benn and Crow, 1990; Scott and Lehman, 1998; Wiersma, Wanderling, Dragomirecka, Ganev, Harrison, An Der Heiden, Nienhuis and Walsh, 2000).

This multi-varied impact of schizophrenia combined with the often dramatic presenting symptoms has given the disorder the reputation of being the prototypical 'serious mental illness'. While this undoubtedly can be justified it has also, at times, led clinicians to engage in practices that disempower sufferers and to do things *to* them rather than *with* them. The current manual is an attempt to integrate the needs of services for rigorous and accountable relapse prevention work with the aim of many clients, that is, to take control over their own life and illness to the greatest extent possible.

In contrast to bipolar disorder, which constitutes the other major category within the severe mental illness diagnoses, schizophrenia has been extensively researched, and the present manual, while based on the original research into relapse prevention in bipolar disorder, uses the extensive research conducted with schizophrenia sufferers and their families. The manual draws on the model set out by Zubin and Spring (1977) and by Nuechterlein and Dawson (1984) when describing the development and relapse into schizophrenic episodes. This model assumes the existence of a latent biological vulnerability in at-risk individuals who relapse when environmental stress occurs to a degree that stretches the sufferers' coping strategies beyond the threshold where they are no longer able to fend off a psychotic relapse. The emphasis on biological/genetic vulnerability *or* stress factors has varied across approaches to treatment, but with approximately 85 per cent of schizophrenic patients not having any discernible family history of the disorder (Wahlberg and Wynne, 2001) the case for arguing that environmental stress factors are important in the expression of psychosis is strong. This in no way implies that medical interventions are not important in the management of psychosis and the current manual will conceptualise medication as a protective factor of great importance for the majority of patients. It is, however, assumed that even optimal medication is rarely a complete answer to an individual's problems as there are likely to be multiple routes and contributing factors to the development of initial symptoms and subsequent relapses into schizophrenia or psychosis generally. Equally, no single psychosocial intervention is likely to offer a resolution to all issues for patients when implemented in isolation and the current intervention is no exception to this rule. What this manual *does* claim to offer is an unthreatening, empowering and collaborative way to engage patients who are often concerned about interacting with services. The manual is not concerned with diagnosis or pathology, but rather with offering practical education and management solutions to problems relating to relapse and worsening symptom profile. The collaborative and non-intrusive nature of the intervention programme, assumed to be related to ease of engagement, is of particular importance as research in recent years has shown that the extent to which an illness goes untreated is related to depression, suicide, later resistance to treatment, use of compulsion and time spent in hospital (Wahlberg and Wynne, 2001). The manual's emphasis on collaboration and the focus on the patient's subjective experience of their symptoms are also thought to prepare the way for engagement in any further, planned cognitive behavioural work. As such, this brief relapse prevention programme should never be used in isolation but rather as a possible first step in the engagement of clients. Thus, the manual is the starting point for a multidisciplinary treatment package although its nature is such that it can, and should, be updated regularly as new information regarding symptoms and coping strategies emerge and the client gains more insight into his or her illness.

Psychological treatment of psychosis, including the development of simple relapse prevention programmes, has often been assumed to be an area requiring extensive training and prior expertise. However, in daily NHS practice, the resources, specialist time and specialist knowledge required to conduct complicated and long-term CBT interventions are often not available. The question then becomes how to reconcile the gap between recommended clinical practice and resources, while also taking account of the fact that the duration of untreated psychosis is a reliable predictor of the long-term outcome for the client, making waiting lists highly unappealing (Eaton, Thara, Federman and Tien, 1998). The answer could be to empower and utilise the skills and experience of personnel that are more readily available in the preparation of further intervention and the 'holding' of clients until the highly skilled CBT practitioners with specialist training in psychosis become available. Thus, the present manual was written with the aim of being useful to non-expert and expert clinicians alike and it is hoped that general practitioners, assistant and trainee psychologists under supervision, as well as more experienced mental health workers will find it a useful instrument when working with client groups experiencing psychosis.

The structure of the manual

Hopelessness is a key predictor of suicidal behaviour, which is well established as a serious problem in schizophrenia (Wiersma, Nienhuis, Slooff and Giel, 1998). Furthermore, hopelessness is likely to come about through the experience, common in psychosis, of having no control over symptoms that repeatedly occur and wreck daily life. Hopelessness is thus linked to a lack of belief in one's future ability to control the various occurring symptoms and to the expectation that these symptoms will make life very difficult or 'hopeless'. The empirical data collected on learned helplessness (Seligman, 1974, 1975) show that this state of mind causes passivity and prevents the individual from discovering that conditions may have changed, so that the perceived helplessness is just and only that: perceived (ibid.). Similarly for hopelessness, and in terms of treatment, an intervention that can increase the perceived control over symptoms is also likely to prompt renewed activity and actual attempts to control the unwanted states or symptoms. When this happens, it is important that clients have access to coping strategies that can disconfirm the perceived reasons to experience hopelessness, which, according to basic behavioural principles, will otherwise be reinforced and become even more entrenched. It is therefore important that clients are given an empowering and non-deterministic understanding of the nature of their relapse into psychosis (this happens in Section 1 of the current treatment) before developing the actual coping strategies (which takes place in Section 2). Further, in order for the treatment to be consolidated and have long-term effects, the social network, which will often have experienced many, seemingly unpredictable relapses, must also be moved to prevent reinforcement or recreation of the learned helplessness and hopelessness. This can be a challenging aspect of any therapeutic effort because people close to individuals with psychosis may, themselves, have internalised a degree of helplessness and hopelessness as a result of seeing past relapses occur outside of the client's or their control (network inclusion skills are developed in Section 3). Equally, families of schizophrenic and other psychosis-prone individuals can, unwittingly, be part of the problem and increase the risk of relapse if they have an habitual style of interaction characterised by criticism, hostility and emotional over-involvement (high expressed emotion). This must be addressed and as psycho-educational (Leff, Kuipers, Berkowitz and Sturgeon, 1985) methods have proven valuable in this regard, inclusion of such elements will form part of the intervention's final sessions. As such, the structure of the manual follows from the fact that an 'empowering' form of psycho-education in relation to psychosis is typically necessary in order for a client to be open to learning relapse prevention and coping strategies. Such strategies are less likely to survive over time if the social network is not included in the reinforcement of a new belief system, which states that at least some control over symptoms can be achieved.

Another key feature of the manual is the development of an individualised handbook, or workbook, for the enhancement of coping. This handbook is developed as an integral and progressive part of the intervention and clients are encouraged to develop and improve on the strategies and information contained in the handbook after the treatment has formally ended. It is hoped that the handbook will become a working document for the client and his or her assigned health worker and that this cooperation around the workbook will provide a sense of taking control over the illness to a higher degree than was previously possible.

In contrast to the previous manual targeting relapse in bipolar disorder specifically (Sorensen, 2005), the current manual is ordered in *sections* rather than *sessions* and it is up to the individual clinician to set the pace of intervention in accordance with the ability of the client. This approach is taken in recognition of the varying levels of functioning within the population of people experiencing psychosis.

Who can conduct the treatment?

Although the manual is formulated with the aim of providing the less experienced health worker with an easy-to-use relapse prevention package, and while the intervention is not designed to delve deeply into psychological problems, it is important to understand that psychosis, and in particular schizophrenia, constitutes serious mental illness that can involve consequences such as suicidal behaviours. As a result, it is up to the clinician responsible for the implementation of the programme to ensure that adequate and appropriate supervision by an experienced and suitably qualified mental health worker is available before embarking on the intervention.

Independent of the therapist's level of expertise, the intervention should be conducted in the spirit of collaboration, with a high degree of shared responsibility for the progression of treatment between the client and the therapist. In relation to this the following techniques and approaches to therapy should be borne in mind as guiding principles with regard to the atmosphere and general style of the intervention:

- *Express empathy*. Listen to the client without criticism, judgement or blame and do your best to listen reflectively and gain a clear understanding of the client's perspective and situation.
- *Do not argue*. Arguing is not productive and challenges to beliefs, including delusions, are best received if they are made with a genuinely open mind and in the spirit of true exploration.
- *Encourage self-efficacy*. The client is likely to need support and affirmation regarding beliefs related to the ability to change and control symptoms. A word of caution: be *realistic*; psychosis is often part of a relapsing disorder and clients are not going to have all their problems solved by any one intervention.
- *Use open-ended questions*. During the discussion sections of the intervention use follow-up questions that cannot easily be answered with a categorical answer (such as 'Yes' or 'No'). This allows the client to engage and think more seriously about the issues.

Using this manual according to your needs and expertise

The conversational style in this manual may seem too prescriptive to the experienced mental health clinician who can stamp his or her own authority on the precise implementation and wording of the intervention. However, the style of writing has been greatly appreciated by less experienced staff using the original manual for bipolar disorder and is a deliberate attempt to make the therapy accessible to assistant psychologists, trainee psychologists, general practitioners, mental health nurses, etc. These members of staff often do much of the day-to-day work with psychotic and at-risk clients, but may not necessarily feel confident in taking control over the management of an intervention programme. As a result, and while this is not advisable, the manual is written in a style that, in theory, would allow a less experienced clinician to simply read it out, word for word, with a client.

The manual is written with individual therapy in mind, but it would be a relatively simple matter to change it to a group format. This would enable the therapist to reach more clients and would allow the group participants to inspire and learn from each other during therapy. If the intervention is adapted to a group format, it is suggested that the approach taken is that of 'individual therapy in a group' and that members of the group are matched for social and cognitive functioning. It is also suggested that the treatment is extended to an appropriate number of sessions in accordance with the needs and abilities of the group members.

Finally, it is also recommended that a general assessment of the client's illness model be conducted before the programme is implemented, as the programme uses terms such as 'relapse' and 'illness' which are usually associated with a medical model of psychosis. During implementation of the programme these terms can usually be substituted by terms such as 'problems' or 'concerns' but the client has to believe that there are 'problems', or he/she needs to have 'concern' to some degree. If the client does not believe that there are any problems of a nature that a professional would typically call psychotic, the present manual would be difficult to implement.

Section 1

Information for the therapist

This section, consisting of the programme's early session(s), is designed to give clients an empowering and non-deterministic understanding of the nature of psychotic relapse whether in the context of schizophrenia or not. The sessions should further serve to familiarise the client with the collaborative therapeutic relationship promoted in this intervention programme. This is achieved via a description of psychosis within a stress-vulnerability framework such as that developed by Zubin and Spring (1977). The session should stress the client's ability to play an active part in managing the disorder and its related problems.

For the therapist it is vital to realise that the first sessions should set up the following sessions in the sense that hope of a realistic nature regarding an increased degree of control over internal, mental states should be instilled. This is a necessary first step in the treatment process, as many clients will come to treatment with past experiences indicating that no such control is possible. The first session should answer the question: "Why should I attempt to learn new behaviours and strategies?" while also providing general information about the nature of psychosis.

Welcome and short statement about the purpose of the treatment

Welcome and thank you for coming. The plan for what we will be doing over the next few sessions includes the development of both your knowledge and your coping strategies in relation to the problems you have been experiencing, which you may understand in one of several ways. During the sessions we will look at what these experiences are, and while you have been referred to this programme with what professionals call psychotic symptoms, you do not need to agree with this term as a true description of the things that are causing you problems; the programme can be helpful independently of the way you understand the issues. We will look at the nature of your particular problems and what they look and feel like. We will discuss and describe your symptoms or experiences of relapsing into a problematic state of mind and we will look in detail at what can trigger the development of such states. This mapping of what is going on when you begin to develop problems will then be related to what might be effective ways for you to cope and live with psychosis or problems that professionals believe are signs of psychosis.

[Note to therapist: if client rejects the term 'psychosis' and prefers another term, this term should be used to replace 'psychosis' and/or 'schizophrenia' in the remaining intervention. Alternatively the simple term 'problems' can be used to signify the psychotic features.]

At the end of the sessions you will leave here with a personal handbook for understanding and coping with the problems you encounter in relation to relapsing or repeating psychosis. This handbook is made up from the worksheets that we will be using in the sessions and will be developed specifically in relation to your particular and individual experiences and needs. The hope is that you will then continue to update and improve on the handbook once the sessions have ended, so that you are always improving your ability to understand and cope with the problems.

Guidelines for the intervention

A   Whilst you have the right to stop participation at any time, it is important that you come to all sessions, as you, and we, will not be able to assess the benefits of the treatment until all the sessions have been completed.
B   My job is to help you plan a way to cope with difficulties, so if anything goes wrong or you have concerns, please let me know before you leave for the day so that we can attempt to deal with them in the appropriate way.
C   [Give any service specific guidelines regarding confidentiality, etc.]

Discussion

Do you have any comments or questions in relation to these guidelines? Do you have any thoughts on further guidelines or rules for the sessions that you would like to include or discuss?

Agenda

My goal for today is to cover and discuss:

1   What is psychosis, what are its causes and influences?
2   In which context does it happen?
3   The discrimination and stigma caused by the diagnosis.
4   For us to get to know each other as we go along.
5   The outline of what we will be doing next time.

1. Client is educated about the spectrum of psychotic symptoms and about what these symptoms can signify

You are here today because, at some point, you have been given a diagnosis that includes some psychotic features, which cause you difficulties. There may be hallucinations in the form of sensing something that others cannot agree is there. This often takes the form of seeing or hearing things that others cannot see or hear. Or you could have delusions, which are unusual beliefs. A typical example of a delusion is to believe that special messages are being delivered to you, but delusions can take many other forms and it is also common to experience extreme suspiciousness or paranoia. These experiences can be both frightening and confusing, but in some cases people report that they can have a pleasant content and function as a comfort in an otherwise confusing time. For instance, when voices are pleasant and comforting they are frequently not seen as a big problem and this may be why some people prefer to think about their experiences as spiritual in nature rather than the medically sounding 'psychosis'.

But most often psychosis *is* a problem for the person with the experience and whatever the exact problem may be, or whatever we decide to call it, psychosis can express itself quite differently from person to person. It is important for you to understand the different ways that psychosis can look to different people and also that you understand how it is related to so-called normal experiences that can have many of the same features. First of all we need to look at some of the characteristic features of psychosis and then we will look at the context in which they occur. Later we will look in much more detail at your particular experiences with psychosis in order to understand precisely what is happening for you, but for now we will just try to get a general feeling for what psychosis is.

So, firstly, what do you understand psychosis to be? [Discuss this informally with the client while expressing empathy with experiences through clarifying questions in an attempt to understand fully what the client is describing. Then complete worksheet 1 (see below) in the handbook and ask the client to relate his or her own experiences to what is on the worksheet. Does this conform to the client's own experience of psychosis?]

Section 1
worksheet 1

Common experiences in psychosis

What is psychosis?

Psychosis is a state of mind that impacts on the way a person experiences the world by changing thinking, feelings and the way he or she understands the world more generally. This can typically involve surprising, and often upsetting, experiences such as hearing, seeing or sensing things that are not there (hallucinations) or believing things that most other people do not think are true (delusions). Psychosis comes in a number of guises and for an individual can contain, more or less, any combination of the features described below.

Emotions: Possibly the most important feature, as psychosis without negative emotions may not be a problem (unless it comes with other difficulties). However, psychosis can have elevated mood features to a degree that normal life becomes impossible (as seen in mania). Psychosis can also be accompanied by extreme sadness, depression, anxiety and/or a 'numb' feeling of detachment from life. Alternatively, moods may shift rapidly and without obvious reason.

Thinking: Thinking is often disturbed in psychosis and it can be difficult to concentrate, as one is easily distracted by many thoughts occurring at once or by a blank and empty sensation in the stream of thoughts. The so-called *thought disorders* signify that psychosis can impact on speaking by making this pressured or forced into a quick and incessant pace, while also causing the person to lose track or to follow many different threads in a conversation all at once. Phenomena such as the experience of having one's thoughts suddenly blocked or removed, or of having them broadcast outside of one's head is not uncommon in some types of psychosis. In general, the effects on thoughts are multiple and varied.

Perception:	The experience or *perception* of the world surrounding a person is always affected in psychosis but this is frequently very difficult to realise while psychotic, even when others may consider this obvious. *Hallucinations* are the classic example of change in perception and are most often experienced in the form of voices. However, hallucinations can occur in any of the five senses. Strictly speaking, *delusions* concern how an individual understands or thinks about what is happening around him or her and are basically strongly held beliefs of an unusual character which most people do not believe to be true. Hallucinations and delusions are often interlinked, in that, a person hearing a voice telling him that someone is about to hurt him may develop a paranoid delusion in the form of believing that others are out to get him when in fact they are not.
Behaviour:	Activity in psychosis can sometimes be reactions to delusions and hallucinations as when a person suddenly leaves home because a delusional belief tells him or her that it is unsafe. Alternatively, a person may become very tired, 'empty' of emotions and lacking in drive and motivation to do or engage with anything. Some people, while psychotic, will also begin to sit in unusual positions and to use gestures or expressions that they otherwise would not use. At times these movements and expressions are experienced as involuntary or outside of the person's control.

Worksheet 1 summarised and introduction of the stress-vulnerability model

As you can see from the worksheet, psychosis is a state of mind that impacts on the way a person experiences the world by changing thinking, feelings and the way he or she behaves in and understands the world more generally. As such, it typically has a big impact on most aspects of life and can fluctuate according to what is going on in your life at a particular time. This is because psychosis is typically sensitive to stress in the sense that stress can make it worse or even be the trigger for a relapse into an episode of psychotic illness. However, the fact that it is so closely related to stress gives us the opportunity to attempt to gain some control over it. We can do this by working out what is stressful for you and by working out what can reduce stress in your life. If we can do that effectively, we will also be able to develop a plan for how to cope and live successfully with psychosis. Remember that this should be the goal and that living a happy and fulfilled life with psychosis is absolutely possible and has been done by many people.

Psychotic illness is often, and typically, a relapsing disorder with episodes that can be more or less severe. So there are usually substantial periods with no significant signs of the problem, which is similar to the way people can live with, say, diabetes, without symptoms of the illness constantly reminding them that they have it. This basically means that the disorder is under control. In diabetes you might be very careful about your diet, or you could be taking insulin regularly, or more likely, you would be doing both. Similarly for psychosis, you can watch out for unhelpful or exaggerated stress, you can take the prescribed medication, or, as is most beneficial for most people, you can do both.

If a diabetic drinks a cola with a lot of sugar in it, or forgets to take his or her insulin, then there will be a relapse and he or she will experience symptoms of diabetes. Similarly, someone with psychosis who experiences excessive and unhelpful stress or stops his or her medication is likely to develop symptoms of the disorder, i.e. to relapse.

Discussion

What sort of experiences have you had in relation to psychosis and stress? If you look back to when it first started, was that a stressful time in any way? Remembering your worst/most powerful experience of psychosis, did you experience a lot of stress in the time leading up to this? [Explore this in detail and discuss how stress can be individually determined in that one person's stress is another person's interesting challenge.]

We have now talked about the main features of psychosis and we have discussed some typical experiences that can go with it. The things we have discussed are summarised in the handbook but we have not yet looked at the different contexts or situations giving rise to psychosis. Some of this information is summarised in a worksheet, which also contains a little more information about psychosis. I suggest that we have a look at this worksheet now and you can tell me if there is anything missing from this in relation to how you have experienced psychosis.

[Go to worksheet 2 and explain/discuss this with the client. This includes adding any situations/contexts to the list if the client identifies that his or her psychosis is unrelated to the list provided or that the list is incomplete. Also, ask the client to tick the boxes next to contexts they believe to be related to their particular psychosis.]

Section 1
worksheet 2

Spectrum of psychotic experiences

Context where psychosis *occurs*	What can typically happen in *the context in question?*	*Is it a problem?*	Tick box if this occurs to you
'Normal' or common situations and states of mind	Around a quarter of all people are said to see things or people that are not there. Hearing voices or one's own thoughts spoken out loud is even more common. Equally, at least half the population believes in things that science would dismiss as 'bizarre'[1]	For some people it is a problem, for others it is not. It is possible that the interpretation that the individual puts on these experiences determines whether it becomes a problem	☐
Shamanistic and other religious experiences	In some cultures and religious communities hearing voices or seeing things that others cannot hear or see is seen as positive	Unlikely to be a problem unless the visions or voices are unpleasant. The social context says that it is a privilege and this is important for how it is experienced	☐

1   For more information see, for instance, Bentall, 2004; Bentall and Slade, 1985; Barrett and Etheridge, 1992, 1993, 1994; Hanssen, Bak, Bijl, Vollebergh and Van Os, 2005; Ross and Joshi, 1992; Tien, 1991.

| Sensory deprivation (participants in research suspended in water tanks or confined to bed) | Experience of visual hallucinations and increased *suggestibility* (i.e. become more likely to believe in unusual things such as psychic or occult phenomena) (Scott, in Slade, 1984; Kingdon and Turkington, 1994) | Most people only last for a short time (a few hours) in water tank sensory deprivation before asking for the experiment to stop. This gives an indication that it is unpleasant. But again this depends greatly on how the individual experiences and perceives the situation | ☐ |
| Physical illnesses/organic psychosis. These 'secondary' psychotic states can arise from illnesses including: brain damage or tumours, epilepsy, certain types of dementia, meningitis, multiple sclerosis, sarcoidosis | Visual and other hallucinations and also delusions can be experienced | Yes. Usually a complication in the treatment of an already distressing illness and distressing in itself | ☐ |

Drugs, LSD, 'magic mushrooms' and other hallucinogens are specifically taken to experience psychosis. Cocaine, amphetamines, anabolic steroids, heroin and cannabis have all been linked to triggering psychosis	Depending on the particular drugs, hallucinations and delusions are relatively common and users can hear voices, become paranoid and aggressive, or can be 'dreamy' and relaxed with somatic/physical hallucinations such as colour vision and changed body sensations	The psychotic features can be the desired effect as in the use of LSD but users can have 'bad trips' which are highly unpleasant. Drugs bring with them many social and personal problems and the psychotic features are highly undesirable for most drug users	☐
Hostage situations (involuntary confinement without social interaction)	Hallucinations are common (Siegel, 1984)	Usually distressing but if kept in isolation for extended periods a voice can be considered 'company' and something to relate to	☐
Bereavement	It is very common to see or hear a recently deceased person if you had a close relationship with that individual	Can be frightening as it is not widely known that this is a common experience but it can also be comforting to feel close to the deceased again	☐
Brief reactive psychosis	Hallucinations and/or delusions that pass after a short period, following a stressful life event (i.e. house move, divorce, becoming homeless, etc.)	Usually distressing for the brief duration of the experience	☐

Severe depression	Hallucinations and/or delusions that can last the duration of the severe depression	Distressing as the content of hallucinations (voices) and delusions are usually similar to the depressive state in that they are negative and harsh towards the sufferer	☐
Bipolar disorder	Hallucinations and delusions can occur in both the manic and the depressed phase of this illness commonly known as 'manic-depression'	Symptoms in the depressed phase are similar to those in severe depression but in the manic phase a person would usually feel grandiose ("I can do everything") or paranoid	☐
Schizophrenia	Full range of psychotic experiences, from lack of initiative to very active engagement and bizarre behaviour in relation to hallucinations and delusions. Thought disorders are also common	Usually has unpleasant features but it is not uncommon to hear people with schizophrenia say that they like the 'company' of their voices	☐

Any other context that you want to include?

2. Client is educated about the high prevalence of psychosis and a discussion about stigma facilitates the therapeutic relationship

Schizophrenia affects about one in every 100 people over their lifetime, which is about the same as the number of people affected by diabetes, and psychosis generally occurs in approximately one in four people and as such is very common. It does not discriminate between genders and it affects people from all walks of life. However, despite the fact that it is a relatively common occurrence, it is rarely discussed openly in the same way as something like diabetes. This can mean that people who have this type of problem can feel lonely and on their own with the problems that the disorder can cause. The reasons why people do not like to talk about having psychosis vary from person to person, but it is common to fear the stigma of being labelled, or to fear discrimination because of a particular diagnosis.

However, it is important to know that lots of people have it and that a likely reason that you probably do not know many people with the diagnosis, outside of any patient groups that you attend, is that most do not discuss the illness openly outside of the family or other very close relationships. It is also important to realise that many people manage the illness well and have fulfilled lives while living with a psychotic disorder.

Discussion

Do you know anyone with schizophrenia or other types of psychosis? How is their life? Have you been discriminated against because of your psychosis? Do you think that it is a good idea to be open about having the diagnosis? Are there situations where you would not tell people and situations where you always would?

3. A multi-model intervention strategy is argued for by presenting causes and influences within the stress-vulnerability model

Questions that many people with psychosis have are: "Why me?" and "What can cause an episode of illness?"

In this treatment I differentiate between the factors that caused the original onset of the disorder, and the factors that influence how the disorder manifests itself later on. The reason for this is that these factors are not always the same.

Genetic factors are thought to play an important role in causing the initial episode of the disorder, so having schizophrenia or another defined psychotic illness in the family appears to make it more likely that certain people will develop such disorders themselves. It is slightly different when we look at subsequent episodes which take place after the initial one because these so-called relapses appear to be heavily influenced by other factors such as stress, sleep disruption, substance abuse, not taking medication, etc. These are all things that we can work at changing if we choose to do so, just like someone with diabetes can change what they eat or whether they take insulin.

Looking at the issues in this way means that psychosis is not just a matter of psychological problems, or just a matter of a chemical imbalance in the brain. In fact it can be both of those things at the same time.

This means that a useful model for helping us to understand relapse in any psychosis-related problem has to take account of both of these aspects and combine them in a sensible manner. In other words, it makes sense to look at the disorder as an interaction between *biological factors*, such as reduction in the effects of chemicals in the brain, *psychological factors*, such as hopes, expectations, predictions and interpretations about things in your life, and *stress factors*, such as having a child that does not sleep through the night, conflict with a partner, a difficult job situation, moving house, financial difficulties, etc.

We all have a certain degree of vulnerability to psychotic episodes at the biochemical level. You might have been born with a tendency for over- or underproduction of certain chemicals that work in the brain to keep psychosis at bay or the nerve cells in your brain might not be using the chemicals in the best way possible.

Much of the time these vulnerabilities will not impact on your day-to-day life. But when you encounter a lot of stress and this rises above a certain threshold, then the vulnerabilities can be expressed as the psychotic features we saw earlier. So the biological vulnerability can impact on your psychological and emotional reactions to the stressful things going on in your life at that particular time. If we take away the stress that triggered the episode, then it is more likely that the biological vulnerability will no longer be expressed and a new psychotic episode will be less likely to take place. We can learn from what has triggered episodes in the past, and thereby start to build up knowledge about the things that stress you in a way that should be avoided because they make it more likely that you will become ill.

Another way of looking at the same relationship between vulnerability and stress is to say that we have to balance our *basic vulnerability* and the *stress* we experience with *protective strategies* that can help us reduce the stress levels and which will allow us to cope better with whatever life throws at us. [Discuss Figure 1.]

Section 1
worksheet 3

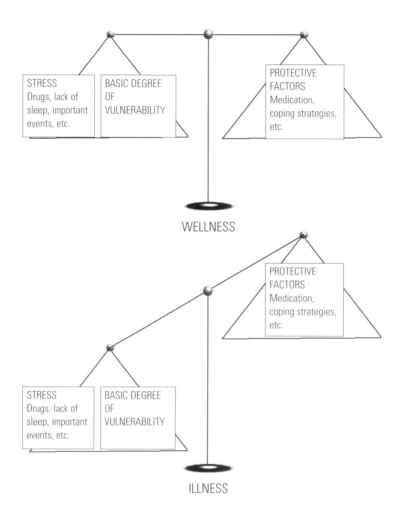

STRESS
Drugs, lack of sleep, important events, etc.

BASIC DEGREE OF VULNERABILITY

PROTECTIVE FACTORS
Medication, coping strategies, etc.

WELLNESS

PROTECTIVE FACTORS
Medication, coping strategies, etc.

STRESS
Drugs, lack of sleep, important events, etc.

BASIC DEGREE OF VULNERABILITY

ILLNESS

Figure 1 *Scales of illness or wellness – a balancing act*

Figure 1 explained

This model shows how someone with a high degree of genetic vulnerability, for example if schizophrenia has run in the family for several generations, would need only a low level of stress to see the scales tip in the direction of illness and for an episode to be triggered. Similarly it shows that someone with very little genetic vulnerability would need to experience more stress to produce an episode.

More importantly for what we are doing here, the model illustrates that there are things we can do to gain some control over the disorder. These are the 'protective factors' shown in the figure. If we get to know what particular stress factors to look out for, it becomes possible to shift the weight of the scales to a more balanced position by avoiding or managing the stress in question.

There are several different things we can do to reduce the risk of relapsing into illness, ranging from the way we work and live our lives generally, to the way we approach medication. These protective factors or strategies are some of the things that we will be looking at during the next sessions.

Discussion

Can you recognise the idea that stress makes it more likely that a relapse will take place? [Note to therapist: exams, job interviews, moving house, etc. are likely situations where relapses may have occurred in the past.] Have you experienced an episode coming out of the blue, without any warning?

Next session

Next time we will begin to focus on your particular problems and psychotic experiences. This will involve an exploration of how you developed the problems and an examination of what they are in more detail. This will then allow us to start looking at what you can expect if a relapse into illness starts to happen again, which in turn will allow us to come up with some suggestions for what you can do to make it less likely to happen. The hope is that this will enhance your ability to manage the problems in a proactive way and therefore increase your ability to control the psychosis.

Section 2

This section is designed to aid the client's awareness of his or her own early signs, symptoms and triggers for an episode of illness. This will enhance the ability to manage the disorder in a proactive and functional manner that is personally meaningful to the individual.

Agenda and aims for session(s) in Section 2

1 Develop a list of signs and symptoms of psychosis individual to the client.
2 Develop a list of triggers for psychosis individual to the client.
3 Develop an individual psychosis profile (thoughts, behaviours and feelings characteristic of the individual client's psychotic episodes).
4 Put the signs and symptoms on a timeline in order to determine at what point in the relapse particular symptoms appear.
5 Determine personal criteria for when to react to changes in the psychosis profile and list the actions to take.

Introduction to today's session

We saw last time that psychosis can be characterised by a number of different features or symptoms that involve quite extensive changes in emotions, thinking and behaviour, compared to what was happening before the psychosis occurred in your life. The fact that psychosis can be very different from person to person reminds us that each person is unique and should be treated as an individual. Understanding how one's own particular illness expresses itself includes being able to recognise the symptoms that form a typical, but individual, pattern and is a first step towards developing coping strategies that can eliminate, or at least limit, the recurrence of episodes of illness. This is very important because even the perfect plan for how to cope and what to do is not very useful if we do not know when to put the plan into action. Today we will begin to develop your personal lists of signs, symptoms and triggers of psychosis. This will then lead us on to finding and describing your individual and unique profile of psychosis, which is made up of the thoughts, behaviours and feelings that go with your particular difficulties. This, in turn, will enable us to develop better criteria for recognising when to react to changes in the symptom profile, and we can then list the actions to take in order to combat the psychosis and also develop a more precise understanding of when certain signs and symptoms appear on the timeline towards relapse.

Discussion

[Have a conversation about the client's experiences before a relapse by focussing on the most recent or 'worst, first or most memorable' relapse. During this discussion the therapist should show an interest in the question of *when* particular signs appeared in relation to others, i.e. "So you stopped going to work *before* hearing voices speaking about you but *after* you had the first anxiety and restlessness?".]

Suggested questions

- What happened last time you were admitted to the ward?
- What was going on in the days leading up to the admission?
- How did you spend your days?
- How did you feel?
- Did you think about anything in particular?
- When did you first notice that things were changing?
- With hindsight can you think even further back in time and see that things were beginning to change even if you did not notice it at the time? [If so, what and when did things start to change?]
- Did it help being in hospital?
- How did you know that things were getting better? [i.e. what changed to tell you that the psychosis was not so strong anymore?].

1. The development of a personal list of symptoms of psychosis and the development of an individual psychosis profile

Thinking back to the last section and the worksheets we considered, it was clear that human experiences, including psychotic ones, are largely made up of the way in which a person experiences his or her own thoughts and feelings, combined with how the person then behaves. So while we know that certain symptoms must be present in order for a diagnosis of, for instance, schizophrenia to be made, the experience of schizophrenia, or any other form of psychosis, can reasonably be summed up by the particular thoughts, feelings and behaviours that characterise the individual illness, which in turn will vary somewhat from person to person. This obviously assumes that the hallucinations and delusions are part of an underlying illness and are not correct representations of the 'real' world even if they can be powerful and convincing and therefore *feel* real at the time. Viewing psychosis in this way implies that delusions and hallucinations are really thought content produced in the mind of the person with psychosis and that they can therefore be seen as thoughts, just like other thoughts that a person may have but with the added twist that these particular thoughts may appear as, for example, voices and strongly held, but incorrect, beliefs or delusions.

Discussion

Thinking back to our last session, what kind of experiences can a person have when he or she is psychotic? And what might he or she do? [Note to therapist: if no examples are generated ask specifically about thoughts, feelings and actions/behaviours relating to the individual client.] Does this general pattern correspond to your particular experiences with psychosis or do you think that your psychoses are different in any way?

[Note to therapist: write down suggestions on a board/flipchart under the headings of: 'Thoughts', 'Feelings' and 'Behaviour'. A category of 'Other' can be added if the client does not see hallucinations, etc. as thoughts. Alternatively, facilitate a discussion about how 'perceptions' (including hallucinations) and/or 'cognitions' (including delusions) can generally be seen as thoughts. A clinical judgement is required in order to determine which model is most beneficial for the individual client, i.e. can a brief corrective discussion on the nature of thoughts and perceptions bring the client to acknowledge the three-factor structure of 'Thoughts', 'Feelings' and 'Behaviour'? Conversely, is the client more likely to need the inclusion of the fourth category of 'Other'?

If the client does not generate a sufficient number of examples, suggest common symptoms (and use your knowledge about the client from the psychiatric file) and carefully check that these are part of the client's experience of psychosis before including them on the list (see Appendix for inspiration with regard to common symptoms).

When a reasonable list has been generated, direct the client's attention to *Section 2 worksheet 1*: *Individual psychosis profile* and ask the client to check off symptoms that represent his or her particular psychotic experiences and to add relevant symptoms not listed in the blank spaces, while checking off the first occurring warning signs of relapse with an 'F'.]

Section 2
worksheet 1

Individual psychosis profile

Tick the symptoms you recognise from your own experience. Put an 'F' by those which you feel are first indications that an episode might be under development.

Thoughts and perceptions:

☐ Difficulties with concentration
☐ Feeling lonely and isolated
☐ Hallucinations or delusions (see worksheet from Section 1)
☐ Persistent thoughts about other people being 'out to get you' or about them disliking you
☐ Suicidal thoughts

Add your own examples:

_____
_____
_____
_____
_____
_____

Feelings:

☐ Drained of energy
☐ Feeling that you are useless to other people
☐ Feeling low/down even when things that should have cheered you up occur
☐ Easily angered and irritable (short fuse)
☐ Lack of self-confidence
☐ Feeling elated and overly happy
☐ Sadness all or most of the time
☐ Appetite gone

Add your own examples:

_____
_____
_____
_____
_____
_____

Behaviours:

- ☐ Eating too much or not enough
- ☐ Sleeping too much or too little
- ☐ Often tearful with no clear reason
- ☐ Must be on the move at all times to combat restlessness
- ☐ Stopping usual activities, being inactive
- ☐ Seeking solitude/wanting to be alone
- ☐ Difficulty starting or completing tasks

Add your own examples:

_____

_____

_____

_____

_____

_____

Immediately after completion of worksheet 1, ask the client to consider worksheet 2A and use the information on worksheet 1 to identify and make more precise the order in which a relapse has happened. [See instructions for completion of worksheet 2A on the worksheet.] It is common for clients to have difficulties remembering the sequence of relapse signs precisely and it is often helpful to direct them to consider their *last*, *first* or *most serious* relapse. It can also be helpful to consult the psychiatric file and to complete worksheet 2A over two sessions in order to allow the client to consult friends and family members who often remember details not retained by the client. Worksheet 2B is a copy of worksheet 2A which is included in the manual and workbook to facilitate and emphasise the importance of continually updating and making improvements to the relapse prevention programme even after the initial intervention has ended. This also applies to the inclusion of multiple copies of other worksheets in the current programme and this logic should be explained to the client who needs to be given a sense of personal 'ownership' and shared responsibility for the psychosocial aspects of relapse prevention.

Section 2
worksheet 2A

Individual psychosis profile in order of occurrence

Look at worksheet 1 and number the individual items that you ticked there below. Do this in order of occurrence when you are becoming psychotic, with the first occurring signs numbered '1', second signs numbered '2', etc. It may be useful to think back to your last or first episode.

You can also ask relatives or professionals who remember or who have access to your file.

Thoughts and perceptions:

☐ Difficulties with concentration
☐ Feeling lonely and isolated
☐ Hallucinations or delusions (see worksheet from Section 1)
☐ Persistent thoughts about other people being 'out to get you' or about them disliking you
☐ Suicidal thoughts

Add your own examples:

_____
_____
_____
_____
_____
_____

Feelings:

☐ Drained of energy
☐ Feeling that you are useless to other people
☐ Feeling low/down even when things that should have cheered you up occur
☐ Easily angered and irritable (short fuse)
☐ Lack of self-confidence
☐ Feeling elated and overly happy
☐ Sadness all or most of the time
☐ Appetite gone

Add your own examples:

_____
_____
_____
_____
_____
_____

Behaviours:

☐ Eating too much or not enough
☐ Sleeping too much or too little
☐ Often tearful with no clear reason
☐ Must be on the move at all times to combat restlessness
☐ Stopping usual activities, being inactive
☐ Seeking solitude/wanting to be alone
☐ Difficulty starting or completing tasks

Add your own examples:

_____
_____
_____
_____
_____
_____

Section 2
worksheet 2B

Individual psychosis profile in order of occurrence

This is a copy of worksheet 2A included here for your convenience so that you can update and change your original individual psychosis profile as you learn more about your signs and symptoms.

Thoughts and perceptions:

☐ Difficulties with concentration
☐ Feeling lonely and isolated
☐ Hallucinations or delusions (see worksheet from Section 1)
☐ Persistent thoughts about other people being 'out to get you' or about them disliking you
☐ Suicidal thoughts

Add your own examples:

_____
_____
_____
_____
_____
_____

Feelings:

☐ Drained of energy
☐ Feeling that you are useless to other people
☐ Feeling low/down even when things that should have cheered you up
   occur
☐ Easily angered and irritable (short fuse)
☐ Lack of self-confidence
☐ Feeling elated and overly happy
☐ Sadness all or most of the time
☐ Appetite gone

Add your own examples:

_____

_____

_____

_____

_____

_____

_____

Behaviours:

☐ Eating too much or not enough
☐ Sleeping too much or too little
☐ Often tearful with no clear reason
☐ Must be on the move at all times to combat restlessness
☐ Stopping usual activities, being inactive
☐ Seeking solitude/wanting to be alone
☐ Difficulty starting or completing tasks

Add your own examples:

_____

_____

_____

_____

_____

_____

_____

When worksheet 2A has been completed the client is directed to worksheet 3A and the example provided is explained.

Say: Looking at worksheet 3 we can see an example of how a relapse can look. You can see that it is shown on a timeline, following the relapse from the first signs to complete relapse and psychotic symptoms. On one side of the timeline we have important life events or things that were happening in this particular person's life at the time of the relapse. This information is used to help remember things that can often be difficult to recall after the event. By putting some context to the time in question we can often start to recall the thoughts and feelings that we experienced at the time and this can then help us to remember what sort of things we were doing. The best way to help our memory is to start at the bottom of the worksheet and work our way up, or back in time, from the actual relapse. So if you look at the example in worksheet 3A you can see that this person was admitted to the hospital ward with hallucinations and delusions in June 2006. If you then look further back to the next memorable event in April 2006 you can see that hallucinations and delusions were also forming quite clearly at that time.

[Note to therapist: work backwards through the timeline example and then summarise by going back through the example, this time chronologically (from November 2005 to mid-June 2006). Following this discussion, a memorable relapse is identified with the client and the timeline provided in worksheet 3B is completed with this information. Typically the best results will be achieved when analysing a recent relapse but the key is to determine the most memorable instance for the individual client and to use this for the exercise. The main reason for summarising the information gained from the previous worksheet in this way, i.e. on a timeline, is that the timeline provides a visual aide to memory and simultaneously makes the information personally meaningful. It is likely that the client will remember new aspects of his or her relapse profile when looking in detail at a relapse timeline. This new knowledge can then be added to the earlier worksheets, thereby demonstrating how improvements to the existing handbook can be made whenever new information is acquired.]

Say: Now that we have looked at the example let us look at worksheet 3B and complete this in relation to your experience with relapse. What is the relapse you remember the best? [Note to therapist: identify this memorable relapse and if the client cannot give a clear indication of a relapse use the last or first example available from the client's history.] We start at the bottom of the worksheet just like we did with the example and we can use worksheet 2 to put some of the experiences you have had onto the timeline.

Helpful explorative questions that can add to the information contained on worksheet 2:

- Tell me what sort of things you were thinking when you were in hospital.
- Tell me what you did in response to your thoughts and feelings while you were in hospital.
- Which of the symptoms from the previous worksheets do you remember most clearly from your time in hospital?
- How long before going into hospital had you had these experiences?
- What was going on at the time? [Ask about world events, sports events, personal events such as birthdays, weddings, job-related issues, etc., depending on the interest and life circumstances of the individual client.]

Section 2
worksheet 3A (example)

Individual psychosis timeline

Important life events	Signs of relapse identified on previous worksheets (worksheets 1 and 2)
Left home to live with Pete (November 2005)	Forgot several things at mum's house, felt a little low in mood
Went on holiday to Spain (Christmas/ New Year 2005/06)	Had no appetite and started to drink more alcohol. Felt very restless, sleep disturbed (nightmares)
Stopped going to work (February 2006)	Asked Pete to stop listening to my private conversations. Stopped trusting Mum to look after Ann (daughter) during the day
Dad's 30th anniversary in the fire service party (March 2006)	Stayed in my bedroom all day
Strike by the fire-fighters (April 2006)	Heard messages about receiving special powers on the radio throughout the day. Waited for 'someone'/the person behind the voice to come at night to give me these powers
Admitted to the ward (mid-June 2006)	Hallucinations (two voices commenting on my behaviour). Delusions (strong belief that I had the power to heal other people's

Relapse complete

Section 2
worksheet 3B

Individual psychosis timeline

Important life events	Signs of relapse identified on previous worksheets (worksheets 1 and 2)

Relapse complete

Section 2
worksheet 3C

Individual psychosis timeline

Important life events	Signs of relapse identified on previous worksheets (worksheets 1 and 2)

Relapse complete

2. The development of a personal list of triggers for relapse into psychosis

Some of the symptoms you have listed on the worksheets used in this part of the programme are the same for most people with psychosis, but it is also important to note that your personal list is a 'cluster' of signs and symptoms that is personal to you, and that you, most likely, have signs or symptoms that someone else with the same diagnosis would never experience as part of their individual psychosis profile.

In the same vein, the symptoms of psychosis can return in several different ways. They can come to you slowly and gradually, increasing in intensity and severity over time, or they can develop quite quickly. It is important to be aware that it is possible to be in the somewhat confusing situation of having conflicting experiences occur at the same time, for instance, sadness and other 'low' experiences while also feeling full of energy or very restless. This can be a particularly difficult state to be in as we are then dealing, not only with the main suffering involved in much psychosis, but also with having to cope with getting mixed messages from mind and body. Nevertheless, this type of experience is not uncommon in problem profiles such as those associated with severe and so-called agitated depression and it can also occur in manic depression, now usually known as bipolar disorder.

Discussion

How have you experienced the occurrence or return of psychosis in the past? Is it a slow and gradual process or is it an overnight, quick relapse development?

Previously I compared psychosis to diabetes where sugar levels can go too high or too low because the body cannot regulate them in the appropriate way. In psychosis it is mood and thoughts that are not being regulated properly. This can lead to mood disturbances as seen in depression and anxiety, and to the various thought disturbances that we have seen in previous worksheets. Both these aspects of the illness will usually fluctuate in their presence and you are likely to have periods of relative stability in both mood and thoughts. However, while some psychotic experiences come once and then never return, the fact that you have been referred to relapse-prevention indicates that you most likely have had some experience of recurrent problems. Is that correct?

[Note to therapist: have a brief discussion about the individual client's relapse history.]

Whether or not you have had many psychotic episodes in your life there is no harm in preparing yourself to be able to spot a new episode on its way. This is because many psychotic illnesses can be of a recurring nature. In fact, it can be said that this recurrence is part of many people's experiences with psychosis and that psychosis is commonly something that can come and go over a lifetime. You could say that instability is a characteristic of the disorder and we know that stress can increase this instability.

Stress can be the result of many things and not just negative things either. You can think of stress as the effect of good or bad life events, so anything that can stimulate your feelings or upset your pattern of daily life can be seen as stress. It is normal for us to respond to good and bad events happening to us with good and bad moods, but with psychosis and schizophrenia you may be more sensitive or vulnerable than most to the stresses of life. Furthermore, if stress triggers an illness episode, the episode can last long after the stress itself has gone. This makes the relationship between the stress and the episode more difficult to see.

Discussion

What kind of stress do you think might bring on psychosis? If you think of your own episodes, can you recall if there was anything stressful going on before you became psychotic? If so, what was it? Have you had any psychoses where you could not see that there were any triggers?

[Note to therapist: list the examples of triggers provided by the client on the board/flipchart, direct the client to *Section 2 worksheet 4,* and facilitate the completion of this worksheet by the client.]

Section 2
worksheet 4

Triggers of my psychosis

Put a mark in the boxes next to stress factors you believe have triggered psychotic episodes for you in the past. Describe the triggers in the space provided and add any that are missing from the list (include any stress factor that you believe could trigger an episode even if this has not occurred to date).

☐ Negative events:

_____

_____

☐ Positive events:

_____

_____

☐ Stop or change to medication
☐ Change in the use of substances (alcohol, cigarettes or drugs)
☐ Moving house
☐ A major loss (job loss, loss of a loved one, etc.):

_____

_____

☐ Relationship breakdown
☐ Conflicts with family, colleagues or others:

_____

_____

☐ Working too hard
☐ Partying too hard
☐ Being on your own too much/feeling lonely
☐ Not getting enough sleep

Add your own examples:

_____

_____

_____

_____

_____

_____

Now you have a list, or a *cluster*, of your personal signs and symptoms of psychosis, which represents your individual psychosis profile and you have ordered this according to the timing of their occurrence and illustrated this on a timeline for purposes of clarity. You also have a personal list of triggers or stressors that you have pinpointed as being involved in bringing about, or contributing to the development of, your psychotic episodes.

3. Determine personal criteria for when to react to changes in the psychosis profile and list the actions to take

On worksheet 1 you have marked the first occurring warning signs of psychosis with an 'F' and on worksheets 2 and 3 you have ordered the signs and symptoms according to timing and occurrence in a relapse. On worksheet 4 you have a list of potential triggers of your psychosis, based on what you know from the past. These lists are unlikely to be complete and you should always attempt to improve and expand on them even after this treatment has finished. Whenever you encounter any of the triggers or warning signs of psychosis that you have listed, you know that you should think about taking action so as not to become psychotic. It is important that you read and learn your triggers as well as the first occurring warning signs so that you are instantly aware when they occur. You should probably take out your handbook and have a look at it on a regular basis. By working at improving your knowledge about your psychosis, over time you will become more and more skilled at determining when a relapse is developing and when a trigger or a potential early sign is simply part of your everyday life and experiences without being directly linked to psychosis. After all, if, for example, sadness and restlessness are early signs of relapse for you, this does not mean that you are relapsing every time you feel a little sad or restless. It does mean, however, that you should be aware and that you should react and seek help if further signs of relapse should appear.

In worksheet 5 some things that you can do to cope with the signs of a relapse are suggested. These are based on the idea that stress can make a full relapse more likely and are therefore designed to reduce such stress.

[Therapist reads through worksheet 5 with client. This includes going through worksheet 6.]

Section 2
worksheet 5

Outline of strategies to combat signs of psychosis

1   Contact your GP or mental health worker to 'touch base' and discuss the best way forward.
2   Check that you have taken your medication. If not, contact your GP or psychiatrist in charge of your medication.
3   Keep up your daily activities but do not go overboard and increase them dramatically.
4   Get your sleep! Good sleep habits should be put in place when you are feeling OK as changes can be difficult to make once psychosis has started (see worksheet 6).
5   Do not use alcohol or drugs. Whatever relief they give you will be short-lived and there is always a price to pay in relation to psychosis.
6   Be part of a support group and contact other members when needing to (go to the meetings even when you lack the motivation to do so).
7   Know what type of activity is right/meaningful for you and implement this.

*See below for inspiration (A–N) with regard to things **to do** and write them here:*

_____

_____

_____

_____

_____

_____

8   Know what is not helpful for you.

*See below for inspiration (A–N) and write things **not to do** here:*

_____

_____

_____

_____

_____

_____

A   Phone a friend and tell them about your concerns.
B   Do some relaxation.
C   Do some exercise (run, walk, yoga, ride your bike, etc).
D   Do a hobby activity.
E   Read a good book.
F   Shopping.
G   Plan a day out for yourself and/or friends.
H   Turn off the TV/radio or use a walkman to block out voices.
I   Talk to your mental health worker.
J   Go and spend time with friends.
K   Do not sit back and become passive.
L   Tell yourself that "this will pass".
M Make sure you get some fresh air every day.
N   Get up in the morning.

Section 2
worksheet 6

How to sleep well

1   Your bedroom should, if possible, only be used for sleeping. If you work, watch TV, eat, etc. in the bedroom, you will get used to being active where you want to sleep and this is counterproductive.
2   Sleep cannot be forced and sometimes it takes time. Relax.
3   Go to bed when you first begin to feel the need. Do not wait as you can start to 'wake up' and become less drowsy again.
4   Keep a routine for getting up and going to bed, and let this be the same on weekends as it is on weekdays. Our brain did not evolve to have a five-day week and does not like change in the sleep pattern from day to day!
5   Your body will only allow so much sleep in any 24-hour period. So, if you sleep or nap during the day, you will find it difficult to sleep at night.
6   Limit the night-time use of alcohol, tobacco and caffeine products to an absolute minimum.
7   Discuss the timing of medication intake with your doctor and let him or her know your concerns about sleep.
8   Exercise is tiring and will help you sleep but not if you do it immediately before going to bed.

Finally

Changes in sleep patterns take time and improvements may not be felt until two to three weeks after implementing the suggested habits and practices. Be patient; it will improve if you follow the above guidelines.

Discussion

If you look at items 7 and 8 on worksheet 5 you can see that they mention things to do and things not to do. From your experience what are the things to do and not to do when at risk of becoming psychotic?

[Note to therapist: write down your own and the client's suggestions on the board/flipchart and direct the client to write the examples in the space provided on the worksheet.]

Now we will look at worksheet 7.
[Read through worksheet 7 with client.]

Section 2
worksheet 7

Plan for when at risk of becoming psychotic

Plan for when at risk of becoming psychotic

1 Have I taken my medication?
2 Am I overdoing the alcohol or am I using drugs?
3 What are the stress factors and triggers encountered and is there a simple way to change them?
4 Carry on with normal activities but do not 'overdo' them.
5 Most important things *to do:*

_____

_____

6 Most important things *not to do:*

_____

_____

7 Contact trusted person:
   Phone: _____ Phone: _____
8 Contact GP or mental health worker:
   Phone: _____ Phone: _____
9 Emergency contact line/crisis line
   Phone: _____

You can see that there is room for the names and phone numbers of people you trust and think would be good to talk to in this type of situation. It is a good idea to put down more than one person in case you are unable to contact a particular person when the need arises. There is also room for you to add the phone numbers of your mental health worker or your GP. These could be important if you are at risk of becoming psychotic. If you have these names and numbers ready please fill them in now. If not, please fill them in as soon as you get home today so as not to forget. You should also write in the most important things *to do* and *not to do*. Have a look at the lists we have completed earlier today, in particular worksheet 5, and write in what you feel is most important to you.

Worksheet 7 constitutes a little card that summarises the most important things for you to remember when at risk of a relapse into psychosis. The card is printed for you [give the client the cut-out card included in the pack and help them complete it] and should be kept with you at all times as it can help to have some simple, written information about what to do if you find yourself in a situation that might trigger a psychotic episode. To have the information in written form can be very useful, even if you are confident that you can easily remember these things, because memory and concentration are unlikely to be at their best when you are at risk of, or even just worried about, becoming psychotic.

Next section

Next time we will begin to look at how the developed strategies can fit into, and be strengthened by, the way you live your life in general, at home and at work. This is an important aspect of how you cope and feel about life in general so we will look at how your psychosis might be experienced by the people around you. We will discuss whether you should tell them about your situation and about your psychosis in particular, and we will discuss what you should tell them if you decide that this is the right thing to do. We will also look at some ways to think about and handle employment and employers to minimise the stress you experience.

[Note to therapist: if the client is not in employment, refer to the possibility of future employment, volunteer work, day-hospital attendance or any other activity that fills a substantial amount of time in the person's life and requires continual commitment.]

So next time we will:

1   Discuss information relating to psychosis for family members. What should they know? Look at common problems arising in the family and in the wider social network as a consequence of psychosis. We will also look at how this can be handled and we will work on some communication techniques that can be helpful in this regard.
2   Finally we will review the handbook and say goodbye.

Section 3

This section is designed to integrate all the illness management strategies developed in the previous sections into the client's social and work-related activities. This includes education about how his or her family might experience psychosis and will also develop communication skills and an individually tailored approach to employment and employers.

[Note to therapist: if the client is not in employment, relate these aspects of the session to the possibility of future employment, volunteering activity, day hospital or any other activity that takes up much of the client's time.]

Agenda and aims for session(s) in Section 3

1 Gain insight into the importance of involving your family in coping
2 Gain insight into adaptive communication skills regarding psychosis
3 Develop a plan for how to manage work situations, including communication with employer

Introduction to today's session

Following an episode of psychosis you will most likely look forward to getting things back to 'normal' with your friends, partner, your wider family and at work. It is, however, important to realise that the experiences of the illness, and of you as a person, may have changed the perception that people around you have.

People are often angry and can blame you for being ill, or they can be extremely worried that you may become ill again and treat you in a way that feels overprotective or even patronising. Your colleagues may not know how to handle the situation and can start distancing themselves from you as a result of fear or misunderstandings about what could cause a relapse. Equally, your employer may think that you are not up to the job and could start marginalising you in the workplace, passing you over for promotion, or start to neglect your professional development. So it is important to work out how to handle these situations and to make the necessary adjustments so that people can see you for who you are and so that you can be an effective person at home and at work.

These are the kind of questions we will be looking at today. If you are not currently working, the part of today's session dealing with work is still relevant to you, as you might take up employment in the future, or you can relate the discussion to other aspects of your life that may be stressful in the same way as employment can be stressful. This could include attending a day-hospital or volunteering on a regular basis as these activities contain many of the same stress factors as working in paid employment.

1. Family members and psychosis: the need for good communication skills

Psychosis often involves some behaviour that can be very difficult to understand from the outside, and from the perspective of a family member an understandable reaction is frustration. For instance, this can take the form of confusion and annoyance: "But *why* could you not get out of bed and eat a little bit of breakfast?" or "But *why* did you blame me for things that have never happened?" It is common for people to become frustrated, not only with you, but also with themselves because they care about you and feel that they should help but do not know how. When people are frustrated and perhaps feel guilty that they are unable to help, they often turn to blaming you for the illness, or to being extremely vigilant with regard to any sign of the illness, which can lead you to feel that you are constantly being watched or treated like an irresponsible child.

Blaming can take several forms but will typically involve criticising you for not getting better, or for not trying hard enough to become and stay better. It can involve name-calling or references to you being a bad person, or it can involve accusations that you are selfish because you, for instance, appear to enjoy having delusions of grandeur and therefore stop taking your medication.

Discussion

Have you ever felt blamed for being ill? If so, what happened? Do you understand why someone could blame you for the illness?

The possibility that some people are so worried about a relapse that they become over-concerned with looking out for signs or symptoms of illness in your everyday behaviour is most often an indication that they care and worry about you. Nevertheless, such concerns can feel like 'nagging' and this is often very stressful for someone in your position. This is because worrying about the illness returning can sometimes cause the people around you to have a tendency to interpret most of the things you say or do in terms of the psychosis. This type of 'over-inclusive' thinking, in relation to the illness and your behaviour, amongst your loved ones, can mean that many of the normal things you do or say are seen as part of a psychotic illness when, in fact, they are really not. For example, if you have had a bad day at work and feel a bit upset about this and your reactions are not taken for what they really are, 'normal', but are seen as a sign of relapse into psychosis, you are likely to feel misunderstood and may be humiliated and this is in itself stressful.

Discussion

Have people around you been worried about relapse to such a degree that they treated you differently or even made you feel like a child? What happened?

The worst-case scenario is that over-inclusive thinking amongst people around you, where much of what you do or say is interpreted as signs that an episode of the illness is about to happen, could actually stress you to a degree that initiates a relapse. If, for example, you are having a good day and feel happy with your achievements at work, you are likely to want to tell people how well you have done, as would most of us. But if you have previously had thoughts or delusions of grandeur during a psychotic state your relatives could take your normal sense of achievement as a sign that you are becoming ill again. This could then make them put pressure on you to seek help and they could 'nag' you and repeatedly ask whether you have taken your medication. This, in turn, could make you angry and irritable, e.g. "Why can I not just be proud of my achievements without being seen as ill? Why do you nag me about my medication all the time?" Your relatives could then see this anger, or irritability, as proof that you are indeed relapsing and they would be even more inclined to ask questions about your medication and about whether you should go and see the mental health worker. The result could be a vicious circle that is very difficult to break, which continues to increase the tension and the stress put on you, possibly with actual psychosis as the final outcome. If this were the case it would confirm your relatives' beliefs, i.e. "Told you, we were right all along when we said that an episode was beginning to take form". This is obviously a negative outcome and could increase the likelihood that your relatives will react in a similar fashion next time they see you happy, angry, sad, talkative, confused and so on without any obvious reason. It is therefore very important that we find a way to break this vicious circle.

Discussion

Can you recognise this pattern? The worst possible outcome is that this type of pressure actually triggers an episode. Do you think that that has ever happened to you?

If you are experiencing one or more of the problems we have discussed so far today, the good news is that we will now look at how they can be addressed.

2. Techniques and strategies for educating family and other important people

The first step is to realise that even if relatives or friends have made an effort to understand and listen to your explanations, have spoken to your GP and your mental health worker and have read up on psychosis and schizophrenia, they can still be unclear about what it really means to have such a disorder and about what the future is likely to hold for you and them. It is very important that you take it upon yourself (or ask for extra help from your mental health worker) to educate close friends and relatives. It is a good idea to do this little by little when you think people are in a receptive mood and you should do this even if you do not think that there are any problems with the level of understanding held by the people around you. We do not know what the future will bring and it is better to discuss these things when you do not have any problems because these conversations will be more difficult during periods of high stress, such as when you are recovering from an episode of the illness. The issues should also be discussed following a relapse and during the recovery period, but it will be easier to talk about these issues if you are simply repeating something that you have already mentioned during a period when you were stable in mood and thoughts and not directly affected by a current relapse.

[Explain worksheet 1. It is suggested that clients photocopy and give worksheet 1 to relatives and other significant people in their lives, and that they make themselves available to answer any questions from significant others arising from the worksheet.]

Section 3
worksheet 1

Brief fact sheet on psychosis for family and friends

What does it mean to have psychosis?

The psychotic experience is characterised by an inability to distinguish between what is real and what is not. This can involve a distortion of perceptions and thoughts, which are commonly known as hallucinations and delusions.

Hallucinations are sensations in one of the five senses, which occur without any external influences or 'trigger'. The most common hallucination is in the sense of hearing and typically takes the form of voices, speaking or whispering in the background. However, hallucinations can occur in any of the senses including taste and smell.

Delusions are strongly held beliefs without foundation in reality or strongly held beliefs that are not widely accepted in the culture within which the person lives. Examples of such beliefs may be:

- The FBI is plotting to harm or kill me
- A computer chip has been implanted in my brain to control my thoughts
- I have special powers and I am a special, chosen person (e.g. President, an alien who has come to save the earth, etc.)
- I am receiving special messages and when certain things happen it has a special meaning that only I can understand (e.g. seeing two planes in the sky means that the stock market is about to crash)

In some forms of psychosis, particularly the type called 'schizophrenia', changes to thought patterns are also common. This can involve difficulties with memory and concentration and it can also be characterised by difficulties with keeping to one topic of conversation at a time. Speaking to someone with this problem can be confusing because of the lack of a cohesive structure to the conversation. This can in part be due to the experiences, sometimes seen in schizophrenia, of having thoughts put into, or taken out of, the head by something or someone external to the person. Equally, at times, a person may have the perception that his or her thoughts are 'broadcast', or heard, outside their head. This can feel very intrusive, as no privacy is possible if all of their thoughts are perceived to be heard by others.

Apart from the somewhat dramatic experience of hallucinations and delusions, which are common in all types of psychoses, another set of symptoms can be seen in the psychotic state known as schizophrenia. If the person you know experiences schizophrenia you might see, in addition to hallucinations and/or delusions, some symptoms that are characterised by the absence of behaviours or experiences. If this is the case for the person close to you, what you may see is that he or she starts to lack motivation, energy and emotion, and they might not move for prolonged periods of time. These signs are called *negative* symptoms and can also consist of withdrawal from social life, mood swings, poor self-care and grooming, and will typically be accompanied by difficulties with functioning at work or school. Negative symptoms are similar to those that you might see if someone is depressed and a trained health professional should be asked to distinguish between the alternative diagnoses associated with the absence of behaviour.

About one in every four people will experience some form of psychotic feature during their lifetime although most will not go on to develop a chronic mental illness as a result. So it is a very common experience and can be seen in everyday misperceptions, for example, 'hearing' someone calling out your name in the street when they did not, or in 'hearing' that the telephone rang when you were in the shower, when in fact it did not.

When psychotic features persist over a prolonged period and when they cause significant disruption to life the diagnosis of schizophrenia is often made. About one in every 100 people has schizophrenia, which is about the same number of people with type I diabetes. So schizophrenia is a fairly common illness.

What causes psychosis?

There are various possible causes for psychosis and it can occur as part of an underlying mental illness such as severe depression, bipolar disorder (formerly known as manic depression) or schizophrenia. It can also come about as a result of drug misuse or can be triggered by a life crisis such as bereavement or another major, traumatic incident.

When looking more specifically at the causes of schizophrenia there is much controversy, but most clinicians and researchers believe that the illness is related to having an imbalance of chemicals in the brain and to the way that brain cells communicate with each other using these chemicals. Having schizophrenia is in no way a choice and it is possible that an individual with the illness has inherited the tendency for the disorder from blood relatives, as genetics also appear to play a part in why people develop the disorder.

Finally, the symptoms a person experiences are also likely to be affected by stress and the things experienced in life more generally, such as sudden changes, being overworked, lack of sleep, being criticised in, and stressed by, family life or other forms of stress. Please note that despite the possible impact that a stressful home life can have, the research literature is clear: *families do not cause schizophrenia.*

How does one recognise psychosis in a person?

What you, as a friend or a relative, may see in a person with psychosis can be varied. It is likely that he or she will display a change in mood and that their behaviours and topics of conversation will change from what is usual for that particular person. However, psychosis can take so many forms that general guidelines, apart from what has been raised in the sections above, are very difficult to specify. As part of the treatment that your friend or relative has received, he or she has developed a better understanding of the personal expression of psychosis that is relevant to him or her and it is possible that you may be able to share this information. As such you can ask to be educated and informed about such aspects as the first signs that a relapse may be occurring and other aspects of the psychosis that you may find interesting and useful. Asking for such information is best done when the person close to you is not in an acute psychosis as, at such times, he or she may be unable to tell you the relevant information due to being in an altered state of mind.

Treatment

Treatment will most likely include one of a range of anti-psychotic drugs prescribed by a psychiatrist and may also involve taking anti-depressants in order to help control both depression and any anxiety symptoms that form part of the individual illness.

It can also be useful for a person with psychosis, and for people close to him or her, to go to a talking therapy, be it family therapy or another form of counselling. Likewise, it can be helpful to belong to a support group of people who understand the issues from personal experience and who can share their knowledge about issues to do with: *stress management, communication skills, effects and side-effects of medication, hints about how to obtain the best possible treatment*, etc.

It is not uncommon for people with psychosis to misuse alcohol or other substances. This is likely to make problems related to the disorder worse and to bring with it its own set of problems. If this is an issue for the person close to you, it may also benefit this person, you and others around him or her, if use is made of a support programme such as Alcoholics Anonymous.

How does prolonged psychosis affect family and social life?

Psychosis is a challenge to relationships that can be met with good communication and emotional support. The illness may affect the ability to relate to others in the family and in the wider social network for periods of time. This is particularly true when the person is experiencing an acute episode of psychosis. It is important to know that relationship problems can be resolved through good communication, support and by working at problems over time. At times it can be helpful to see a family/couples therapist or to join a family support group in order to get a new or different perspective on the issues important to coping and general harmony in the family and wider social network.

Future prospects

The prognosis for any individual with psychosis is hard to make but it is noted that even among those with schizophrenia, the condition usually considered to be the most severe mental illness, roughly up to two-thirds of individuals make a partial or complete recovery after receiving the diagnosis.

However, it is also worth being aware that it is not uncommon for a person with schizophrenia to contemplate suicide, or actually attempt to take his or her own life, which illustrates that schizophrenia and other severe psychotic states (mainly bipolar disorder and severe depression) need to be managed well as suicidal thoughts will most often be related to being psychotic or low in mood.

The nature of psychosis is such that a person with this type of diagnosis is likely to have ups and downs in the coming years, but that does not mean that there is any reason to lose hope for the future.

With the help of medication, therapy and generally supportive surroundings, fluctuations in mental state can occur less often and become less pronounced.

With help and support it is very possible to manage the disorder, go after and achieve regular goals in life just like any other person and to have a fulfilled family, social and work life in the years to come.

It is important to develop a relaxed, but precise way of talking about the disorder with your family and other people who are close to you. Different ways of discussing and speaking about the things that someone has experienced in relation to your symptoms and behaviours when you were ill can indicate different beliefs about what causes you to act in a certain way. This is very important because it is much easier for your partner or other family members to be understanding and supportive of you if they believe, for example, that your extreme impatience or angry outbursts are the results of an illness phase, rather than the results of you changing into a grumpy or even aggressive person in general. Similarly, they should be helped to understand that the illness can put you in a depressed mood or make it difficult for you to concentrate on and remember what they are saying to you, without you having become insensitive or permanently 'miserable'. So, it is clearly important to pay attention to the way people around you speak about your behaviour when ill, as a tendency to blame or criticise you for being ill could point to a lack of understanding and knowledge on the part of others when it comes to your illness.

Discussion

Do you feel that your relatives have an adequate understanding of the type of psychosis you experience or do you need to educate them about it?

[Note to therapist: if the client is a parent also ask and discuss: do you think that a special effort should be made to give your children an understanding of these issues? How should this be done? What are some good terms to use with children when describing what it is like to be psychotic? (imagined/wrong ideas, etc. rather than delusions, and "I thought I could hear things but there was in fact nothing there" rather than hallucinations).]

3. Communication skills

The ability to communicate in an effective way with the people around you is linked to good coping with psychosis and with general well-being for you and them. The skills we will look at now are very important, and you need to practise them on a regular basis, preferably when you are well, unstressed and feeling stable in mood, as this makes them easier to use when you are at risk of becoming ill and need them most.

4. Attentive Engagement (AE)

When you are under a great deal of stress or pressure you will most likely find it difficult to pay attention to the problems of others, even when they are related to people who are important to you, such as family members or close friends. However, when you feel stressed it is also likely that the important people in your life experience some of this stress and that they feel a need for your support. If you are perceived to be unwilling to give this support, to at least some degree, it then becomes more likely that the people you rely on for support will find it harder and less appealing to do some of the things that interfere with their life, but which will aid your recovery. For example, they might not stop putting you under pressure to go to a play or a film that they have been looking forward to, but which could be over-stimulating or even feed your potential delusions if you are experiencing some of the first signs of a relapse.

In other words, they might 'force' their needs through if you are not seen to be responding and paying attention to the needs that they are expressing. Similarly, they are more likely to criticise you in a manner that can be stressful to you if they do not feel that you are taking adequate account of their concerns, wants and needs to the best of your ability when you are able to do so.

This illustrates why it is important for your illness management to help your relatives handle their anger or frustration by listening and explicitly showing an understanding of their point of view. When coming out of an episode of the illness, or when feeling under pressure generally, this can sound like a very daunting task, but much can be achieved by relatively simple and fairly undemanding means. This is because your relatives and friends are, most likely, looking for understanding and a reasonable level of attention to their needs, rather than for you to solve their problems or for you to be very active in what you do together. Therefore, what is required is an attentive engagement with what is going on for the people around you. This requires you to take time to listen and to make sure you fully understand what is going on, while also showing that you are making this effort. In the past much attention has been given to what has been called 'active or reflective listening' which can be a useful technique for showing that you care about what a speaker is saying. You can obtain good reading material on this subject if you are interested in reading more.

[Note to therapist: if the client wants more information on active listening techniques give relevant references, such as Miklowitz and Goldstein (1997).]

However, in this programme what is called Attentive Engagement (AE) broadens the definition of good communication from focussing on listening to also taking account of how we express ourselves. AE stresses that the context and the whole set of communication tools at our disposal are important and include body language and how we place ourselves in relation to the person we are attending to as important components of 'good' communication.

[Go through worksheet 2 with client.]

Section 3
worksheet 2

Attentive Engagement

1 *Get your priorities straight.* If someone on whom you rely for support is asking you to attend to his or her concerns you should have a *very* good reason not to oblige.

2 *Indicate that you will give this moment and their concerns your full attention.* This should be done in a clear manner by, for example, sitting down or suggesting that you should both sit down. This simple move shows that you are not about to leave and that this conversation is important to you.

3 *Use open body language.* For example, do not cross your arms or 'square up' by sitting too close with shoulders directly forward. This can come across as being defensive or aggressive. Let your arms rest alongside your body/in your lap and sit a little sideways to the person you are speaking to. Only look away from the other person to aid a comfortable flow to the conversation, or if you are feeling uncomfortable with the eye contact, otherwise look at them with interest in what is being said.

4 *Check and ensure you understand what is said.* Engage and pay attention while making sure that you show that you are engaged by asking questions to clarify and fully understand what the other person is feeling, believing and needing from you. This is not a time for debate. It is a time for you to understand the other person.

5 *Speak less, understand more.* Make sure you speak far less than the other person.

Example of attentive engagement

Person A: "I know that this is a bad time and that you need to go out, but I really need to get our holiday sorted."

Person B [giving top priority to person A's concerns]: "OK, I don't have to leave just yet so let's talk about it, but do you mind if I make us a coffee? Let's sit down in the kitchen. It's a better place to talk."

Person A: "No problem, but I need some answers. I have to book time off from work. Everyone else is booking their holidays and if we don't get this sorted soon we won't be able to go anywhere. I need to know now! No more excuses."

[A and B sit down in kitchen]

Person B: "Fair enough, you're annoyed with me. You think I can't commit and am not paying attention. Am I right? Is that how you feel?"

Person A: "Yes, and I can feel myself becoming annoyed with you again now, because I have already asked you a million times about this holiday."

Person B: "Yes, I can see that it must be annoying. Did you think that we would not get around to discussing it at all?"

Person A: "I just get so frustrated, angry and worried about whether we can do things like a normal couple. And it concerns me to think about a future where little things like this are always going to be a problem."

Person B: "I can understand why you are concerned. Is it only the holiday? Or is it more general than that? I really want to know what you are thinking and feeling about these things so that we can try and plan a way out of it."

[Please note that this particular conversation may seem artificial to you especially when written down, as above. You need to develop and use your own words and style of Attentive Engagement. Remember: practice makes perfect.]

Discussion

Any questions or comments about AE?

In AE the focus is very much on the needs and feelings of the people who are important to you but this does not mean that, at other times, you should not ask for help or make sure that they understand how their behaviour can be more or less helpful to your coping. Once again the people close to you need to be educated about helpful and less helpful ways of interaction with you when you experience psychosis and psychosis-related features, such as those occurring as the early stages of a relapse. In order to aid their education you can photocopy worksheet 3 *Attentive Engagement for family members and friends* and give this to the people you believe could benefit from such information.

[Note to therapist: read through worksheet 3 with the client and check for understanding. Also, consider if particular relatives or friends could benefit from taking part in a session focussing on communication and education about the client's particular psychotic disorder. This type of intervention can often initiate a more open and helpful style of communication without the problematic tendency to criticise and be over-involved in the psychotic person's life which many relatives will, understandably, otherwise engage in.]

Section 3
worksheet 3

Attentive Engagement for family members and friends

When someone close to you experiences symptoms associated with schizophrenia or another type of psychosis this is likely to be a stress factor for everyone involved and not just for the person experiencing the symptoms. You should ask for advice and information from the professionals involved in the care of the person close to you in order to understand more about the issues faced and in order to understand more about the *dos and don'ts* of relating to someone with these problems. However, there are some relatively simple strategies that you can try to incorporate into your interaction with the person experiencing psychosis.

When the person approaches you to discuss things that concern or preoccupy him or her:

1   *Indicate that you will give this moment and their concerns your full attention.* This should be done in a clear manner, for example, by sitting down or suggesting that both of you sit down. This simple move shows that you are not about to leave and that this conversation is important to you. If you do not have time at that precise moment, make a firm commitment to a particular time when the issues can be discussed, and stick to it.

2   *Try to simplify the conversation.* This can be done by only asking one question at a time, only making one request at a time and by making a conscious effort to be clear in your statements. Keep things brief and clear, and, most importantly, do not lose your temper or start criticising or yelling at the other person. Remember that a likely cause of misunderstandings or inability to understand what you are saying is the illness, not deliberate obstruction.

3   *Use open body language.* For example, do not cross your arms or 'square up' by sitting too close with shoulders directly forward. This can come across as being defensive or aggressive. Let your arms rest alongside your body/in your lap and sit sideways, facing in the same direction as the person you are speaking to. Only look the person in the eye to aid the flow of conversation. Often a person with psychosis (in particular the paranoid variant) will not cope well with direct eye contact, so therefore look elsewhere.

4   *Check and ensure you understand what is said.* Engage and pay attention while making sure that you *show* that you are engaged by asking questions to clarify and fully understand what the other person is feeling, believing and needing from you. This may not be a time for debate and often what is needed is for you to show an interest in understanding the other person's point of view and for you to recognise the feelings/emotions involved, whether you agree or disagree with the content of what is said.

5   *Speak less, understand more.* Your engagement with the other person should be as positive as possible. Critical or 'domineering' comments or attempts to control the conversation can be extremely stressful and hurtful for a psychotic person. If, for example, you are tired and/or irritable, it is probably better to arrange the conversation for another time. In general the goal should be to help the person feel understood rather than to make him or her see the realities in the way you do. More often than not, arguing and debating psychotic beliefs will make them even stronger in the person expressing (and being 'forced' to defend) them.

6   *Do not argue.* It is better to leave a subject alone than to attempt to rationalise with a psychotic person. This does not mean that you should agree with delusional thoughts; it simply means that it is better to focus on giving emotional support to the person who may be stressed by both real and psychotic factors. If you help to reduce the real-life stress factors (housing, paying bills, looking after children, access to treatment, school or work problems, etc.) you are likely to fight the psychosis far better than if you take on the psychotic features directly. This is because a direct challenge to delusional thoughts is actually likely to strengthen the thoughts in question.

Some of the principles from AE also apply when you want people to listen to you. For instance, if you want someone to change their behaviour in any way, it is important that you first think about what the situation would look like from their perspective and that you are willing to listen to their perspective. This attitude will make it more likely that they will listen to you and will improve the chance that they will be willing to change the behaviour in question. It is also very important that you focus on your goal rather than on what you feel is wrong with a given behaviour. In fact, if you criticise someone they are more likely to continue the criticised behaviour than if you had said nothing at all!

Discussion

Do you agree that change seldom comes as a result of criticism? How do you react if people criticise you? Do you tend to change the criticised behaviour?

The alternative to criticising is to ask for change by informing someone what you would like to see. This is much more effective as it makes it clear what you would like to see without making a problem out of what is going on at present.

To illustrate this point I wonder which of these statements, designed to change someone's tendency to be over-inclusive when psychosis occurs, you think is more likely to produce the desired result. [Read out the following two statements or, if necessary, write them on the board/ flipchart:]

"I'm really annoyed that we can't have a simple conversation about my future without you bringing up my illness! Why can't you just see that I don't need this and let me get on with my life?"

or

"I understand that you are concerned about my problems but please try to remember that it's very important to me that I can talk about and plan my future just like any other person. After all, we could all get ill."

Discussion

Which one of these statements do you think is most likely to produce the desired result? Why?

[Note to therapist: stating something in a positive manner makes it much easier to accept.]

This type of positive communication is a skill that needs to be practised, but you will find that the more you practise the more natural it becomes. This is something that you should be aiming for, because if it is not part of your normal way of speaking, then it is unlikely to happen when you are under pressure and need it the most. So again, the lesson is to practise when you are feeling good and when there is no tension in the air. It might feel a bit artificial at first, but this will pass once you feel the benefits of this type of communication.

Discussion

Can you recognise from relationships with family members or friends that criticising is often met with defensiveness? Would it be a good idea to involve your family or friends in practising the more positive types of communication?

5. Managing psychosis at work

In order to be successful at work and in other regular activities that can be equally demanding, it is obviously very important to work at maintaining a stable mindset and a stable mood. This will help you to offer an employer what they are looking for, i.e. effective and reliable employees. The same applies if you are attending a day-hospital or doing another regular activity that at times can seem demanding but which ultimately is in your interest and which will benefit you in the long term. This can be seen as another good reason to take medication on a regular basis. It is also essential to realise that the degree of support within the work environment, and the manner in which you approach work and the workplace itself, are important factors in relation to your stability of mood and mind. The key issues then become how you manage to find the right balance between having an interesting job that challenges you in the way you want it to, and keeping work hours, general stimulation and stress levels at a level that does not, directly or indirectly, cause an illness episode to occur or to become worse.

Discussion

Do you think that having psychosis affects your employment? In what way has that happened?

A situation where it is often a good idea to be extra vigilant about a possible relapse is when you start a new job or return to your job after an illness episode. In this situation we often want to impress our employers, and show them that we can offer the company something important despite having an illness. This can result in a feeling of needing to over-achieve at work, sometimes even to a degree where you might feel 'driven' or compulsive about your work. This can, in turn, lead to you feeling down and tired at the end of the working day, and can also result in disturbed sleep patterns, with little sleep during the week and then many hours of sleep at the weekend.

One of the things worth thinking about in relation to your daily activities at work is that you *can* have a fulfilling work life, but it probably needs to be managed more carefully than if you did not have a relatively high degree of vulnerability to psychosis.

Discussion

What are the things that need managing for you with regard to work and the ability to maintain stability of the illness?

Some of the things that often need to be considered are:

- The job itself (what are you doing and could/should this be done differently?)
- The work setting
- Your employer (he or she can also play an important part in maintaining wellness)

To help avoid the stress and trigger factors that we have discussed during the last few sessions, you should think carefully before taking up any job that includes shifting patterns (such as day work one week and night-time work the next); jobs with frequent sudden/unscheduled social stimulation and demands for socialisation; jobs with little 'off-time' or which include a permanent on-call element; jobs with frequent travel across time zones or a large degree of interpersonal stress. This does not mean that you cannot work in an environment where these stress factors exist, just that they need to be managed extra carefully and that some arrangement may need to be negotiated with your employer.

In order to come to an agreement with your employer, you first need to make sure that they know that you have a psychotic illness.

Discussion

Can you give me some reasons why not to tell your employer about your condition? Can you give me some reasons why it would be a good idea to tell your employer? Could you use worksheet 1 to tell your employer about the issues?

[Note to therapist: go through worksheet 4 and ask the client if, and when, they are going to approach their employer. If they are not in employment, discuss which of the changes/adjustments they can make in their daily activities.]

Section 3
worksheet 4

Managing the workplace

- Tick the box if you think this would benefit you in your current job/daily activity
- Put an 'E' next to the box if you believe your employer would agree to it
- Put an 'A' next to the box if you intend to approach your employer about this

Work structure:

☐ Working same hours every week
☐ Working from home (fully or partly)
☐ Saying no to overtime
☐ Part-time or reduced hours rather than full-time employment
☐ Avoiding shift work

Add your own examples:

_____
_____
_____
_____
_____
_____

Strategies with potential benefit for stability in illness:

☐ Working with others, so blame and credit will be shared and not down to you alone
☐ Working in a low stimuli and inviting environment (minimise noise and work in an uncrowded, uncluttered room, etc.)
☐ Saying no to activities or aspects of the job that have acted as triggers for illness episodes in the past (check lists from Sections 2 and 3)
☐ Taking regular and frequent breaks during the day

Add your own examples:

_____
_____
_____
_____
_____
_____

When not able to work:

☐ Being allowed the freedom to work back time used for mental health appointments at another time

☐ Being allowed to leave work when you spot the signs of a relapse emerging

Add your own examples:

_____

_____

_____

_____

_____

_____

Communication with your employer:

☐ Knowing what your employer is thinking about your job performance

☐ Knowing what your employer is thinking about psychosis

☐ Having an appraisal system based on general performance rather than on punctuality and number of hours completed every month

Add your own examples:

_____

_____

_____

_____

_____

_____

'A's	Date when I will approach my employer
_____	_____
_____	_____
_____	_____
_____	_____
_____	_____
_____	_____

End of treatment

Over the last few weeks you have developed an individualised plan for coping with the particular type of psychotic problems that you live with. You have built up an individual handbook for how to deal with difficult issues such as situations where you notice triggers of a relapse into illness, or where you spot the first signs that an episode of psychosis might be happening. You have a super-concise version of what to do in such situations on a card that you can carry with you everywhere. You have also looked at some of the difficulties that may arise in family and work aspects of life, and have material to share with family members in order to educate them about the disorder and about the things that you might find challenging. This includes some strategies to improve the way you speak to the people close to you about the illness. You have also developed a plan for the things you would like to see improved at work, or alternatively, a list of things that you will think about if you take up employment in the future.

Remember that many of the skills we have talked about are things that benefit from practice, so read your handbook often and try to implement the things that you have decided would benefit you. Practice makes perfect so do not despair if you do not get everything right the first time. No one does.

Before we look through the handbook and remind ourselves what is included in it, do you have any questions?

[Note to therapist: if a booster session is planned this will be set up for two to three months post treatment.]

[Note to therapist: go through the handbook and address any problems in understanding, whilst emphasising that the handbook should be updated and improved on by the client following treatment and when he or she thinks of more things to include.]

Appendix

Signs of psychosis from first relapse to fully developed psychosis

- Hopeless and helpless feelings
- Feelings of being no use to anyone
- Stopped caring about daily life
- Sleep disturbance
- Thinking people are against you
- No energy
- Sad and/or anxious
- Irritable and short-fused
- Feeling strong and powerful
- Feeling guilty without any reasonable cause (free-floating guilt)
- Dislike of oneself or lack of self-esteem
- Concentration difficulties
- Feeling lack of trust in others
- Lost trust in others
- Feeling of being controlled from external source
- Dislike of socialising
- Seeking solitude
- Being indecisive
- Hearing personal communication via radio or TV
- Feeling that others can read your mind or that you can read theirs
- Feeling restless
- Loss of emotions ('hollow'/'empty')
- Extremely tired
- Loss of interest in own appearance
- Motivation to do anything has gone
- Feeling slowed down
- Thoughts and words get confused and unusual words 'sneak' into what you say
- Neglect personal hygiene
- Talking to self or laughing to self
- Senses seem sharper
- Having strange ideas/thoughts
- Hearing voices
- Tactile hallucinations
- Paranoid
- Feeling like a child that cannot impact on own life
- Feeling that others would be better off if you did not exist
- Preoccupied with spiritual or esoteric things
- Believing that others are out to get you (paranoid)
- Believing that you have special powers
- Change in eating patterns
- Having visions (visual hallucinations)
- Thoughts of being dead or unreal

References

American Psychiatric Association. *Diagnostic and statistical manual of mental disorders* (4th ed.), Washington DC, American Psychiatric Association, 1994

Barrett, T.R. and Etheridge, J.B. 'Verbal hallucinations in normals: I. People who hear voices', *Applied Cognitive Psychology*, Vol. 6, 1992, pp. 379–387

Barrett, T.R. and Etheridge, J.B. 'Verbal hallucinations in normals: II. Self-reported imagery vividness', *Personality and Individual Differences*, Vol. 15, 1993, pp. 61–67

Barrett, T.R. and Etheridge, J.B. 'Verbal hallucinations in normals: III. Dysfunctional personality correlates', *Personality and Individual Differences*, Vol. 16, 1994, pp. 57–62

Bentall, R.P. *Madness explained. Psychosis and human nature*, London, Penguin Books, 2004

Bentall, R.P. and Slade, P.D. 'Reliability of a measure of disposition towards hallucinations', *Personality and Individual Differences*, Vol. 6, 1985, pp. 527–529

Blanchard, J.J., Brown, S.A., Horan, W.P. and Sherwood, A.R. 'Substance use disorders in schizophrenia: Review, integration and a proposed model', *Clinical Psychology Review*, Vol. 20, 2000, pp. 207–234

Eaton, W., Thara, R., Federman, E. and Tien, A. 'Remission and relapse in schizophrenia: the Madras Longitudinal Study', *The Journal of Nervous and Mental Disease*, Vol. 186 (6), 1998, pp. 357–363

Hanssen, M., Bak, M., Bijl, R., Vollebergh, W. and Van Os, J. 'The incidence and outcome of subclinical psychotic experiences in the general population', *British Journal of Clinical Psychology*, Vol. 44, 2005, pp. 181–191

Hogarty, G.E. and Flesher, S. 'Practice principles of cognitive enhancement therapy for schizophrenia', *Schizophrenia Bulletin*, Vol. 25, 1999, pp. 693–708

Johnstone, E.C., MacMillan, J.F., Frith, C.D., Benn, D.K. and Crow, T.J. 'Further investigation of the predictors of outcome following the first schizophrenic episode', *British Journal of Psychiatry*, Vol. 157, 1990, pp. 182–189

Kingdon, D.G. and Turkington, D. *Cognitive-Behavioural Therapy of Schizophrenia*, New York, Guilford Press, 1994

Leff, J., Kuipers, L., Berkowitz, R. and Sturgeon, D. 'A controlled trial of social intervention in the families of schizophrenic patients: two year follow-up', *British Journal of Psychiatry*, Vol. 146, 1985, pp. 594–600

Miklowitz, D.J. and Goldstein, M.J. *Bipolar disorder: A family-focused treatment approach*, New York, Guilford Press, 1997

Nuechterlein, K.H. and Dawson, M.E. 'A heuristic vulnerability/stress model of schizophrenic episodes', *Schizophrenia Bulletin*, Vol. 10 (2), 1984, pp. 300–312

Penn, D.L., Mueser, K.T., Spaulding, W., Hope, D.A. and Reed, D. 'Information processing and social competence in chronic schizophrenia', *Schizophrenia Bulletin*, Vol. 21, 1995, pp. 269–281

Rosenfarb, I.S., Nuechterlein, K.H., Goldstein, M.J. and Subotnik, K.L. 'Neurocognitive vulnerability, interpersonal criticism, and the emergence of unusual thinking by schizophrenic patients during family transitions', *Archives of General Psychiatry*, Vol. 57, 2000, pp. 1174–1179

Ross, C.A. and Joshi, S. 'Paranormal experiences in the general population', *The Journal of Nervous and Mental Disease*, Vol. 180, 1992, pp. 357–361

Scott, J.E. and Lehman, A.F. 'Social functioning in the community' in Mueser, K.T. and Terrier, N. (eds.), *Handbook of social functioning in schizophrenia*, Boston, Allyn & Bacon, 1998, pp. 1–19

Seligman, M.E.P. 'Depression and learned helplessness' in Friedman, R.J. and Katz, M.M. (eds.), *The psychology of depression: Contemporary theory and research*, New York, Wiley, 1974

Seligman, M.E.P. *Helplessness: On depression, development and death*, San Francisco, Freeman Publications, 1975

Siegel, R.K. 'Hostage hallucinations: Visual imagery induced by isolation and life-threatening stress', *The Journal of Nervous and Mental Disease*, Vol. 5, 1984, pp. 264–272

Slade, P.D. 'Sensory deprivation and clinical psychiatry', *British Journal of Hospital Medicine*, Vol. 32, 1984, pp. 256–260

Sorensen, J. *Relapse prevention in bipolar disorder. A treatment manual and workbook for therapist and client*, Hatfield, University of Hertfordshire Press, 2005

Sorensen, J., Done, D.J. and Rhodes, J. 'The development and evaluation of a novel, brief psycho-educational and cognitive therapy for bipolar disorder: The Sorensen Therapy for Instability in Mood', *Behavioural and Cognitive Psychotherapy* (submitted)

Tien, A.Y. 'Distribution of hallucinations in the population', *Social Psychiatry and Psychiatric Epidemiology*, Vol. 26, 1991, pp. 287–292

Tsuang, M.T., Wollson, R.F. and Fleming, J.A. 'Premature deaths in schizophrenia and affective disorders. An analysis of survival curves and variables affecting the shortened survival', *Archives of General Psychiatry*, Vol. 37, 1980, pp. 979–983

Wahlberg, K-E. and Wynne, L.C. 'Possibilities for prevention of schizophrenia. Suggestions from research on geno-type-environment interaction', *International Journal of Mental Health*, Vol. 30 (1), 2001, pp. 91–103

Wiersma, D., Nienhuis, F.J., Slooff, C.J. and Giel, R. 'Natural course of schizophrenic disorders: a 15-year follow-up of a Dutch incidence cohort', *Schizophrenia Bulletin*, Vol. 24, 1998, pp. 75–85

Wiersma, D., Wanderling, J., Dragomirecka, E., Ganev, K., Harrison, G., An Der Heiden, W., Nienhuis, F.J. and Walsh, D. 'Social disability in Schizophrenia: its development and prediction over 15 years in incidence cohorts in six European centres', *Psychological Medicine*, Vol. 30, 2000, pp. 1155–1167

Zubin, J. and Spring, B. 'Vulnerability – a new view of schizophrenia', *Journal of Abnormal Psychology*, Vol. 86 (2), 1977, pp. 103–126